MUSIC WITH THE BLUES

CW01080549

MUMS WITH THE BLUES

Dr Trevor Smith

M.A., M.B., B.Chir., D.P.M., M.F.Hom.

Insight Editions
Romsey, Hants
England

WARNING

The contents of this volume are for general interest only and individual persons should always consult their medical adviser about a particular problem or before stopping or changing an existing treatment.

Insight Editions,
Romsey, Hants.,
England.

Published by Insight Editions 2001

British Library Cataloguing in Publication Data

A catalogue record of this book is available from the British Library.

ISBN 0946670 23 4

Printed and bound in Great Britain by Biddles Ltd
www.biddles.co.uk

A SIMPLE BOOK FOR MUMS WITH THE BLUES

FOREWORD

This little book is written for mums of all ages to give a clearer understanding of some of the underlying causes for the 'blues' and a practical approach towards resolving them. Although these vary with each individual mum and include hormonal imbalance or allergy, for many, there is an emotional factor in terms of attitudes, perceptions and understanding, which needs to be thought about and dealt with.

Following the birth, most mums get depressed at some time. It is the norm and not something a mum should become worried or feel guilty about. Feelings of despair, self-reproach and self-pity are just some of the feelings which may develop and cause blockage. The author suggests that mums experiment much more, are prepared to break the rules they set themselves, deal with things differently and in a more direct, straightforward, simple way. She is encouraged to think the unthinkable, to take risks, to make moves, to look again at the many different facets of her being but especially to value herself more.

Once the mum can see a problem area in a different light and from a different angle, she can get a new perspective and begin to see more clearly why she is depressed and feels different within herself. Then she can start to make changes, avoid set ways of thinking, being and doing and take more charge of her life-style and feelings.

The first section is written for young mums. The sections are graded from the most mild 'down in the dumps' feeling, to the terrors and fears of a severe puerperal depression.

Most will not experience severe symptoms but for those who do, a practical approach to lessen their impact and feelings of devastation is included.

A second section is specifically written for husbands and partners. Men often feel threatened by or at a loss to know how best to understand, comfort and respond to a depressed mum, who may be remote or irritable. The relationship of the couple is pivotal to how long the feelings last and how quickly they are resolved. If a mum feels she is driving her partner away or is unable to respond in a happy positive way, this can also intensify feelings of guilt and inadequacy.

A third section is written for the mature mum with the 'blues'. Problems may occur within her own relationship, leading to arguments, lack of support, withdrawal, feelings of panic or alienation. Divorce or the death of a partner, can be catastrophic if the mum has always been in a secondary or dependent role. Problems also arise when the children marry and she does not approve of the partner, or if they have marital problems and divorce, causing her to re-think her own life-style and relationships and come to terms with her son or daughter's new partner.

A final section gives suggestions for complementary therapy and a list of safe remedies you can take, whatever your age and whether you are pregnant or nursing the baby.

This is not a book to read through quickly. Only attempt to read one or two pages a day, not more. Think about each page and see how it relates to you. Don't read it for entertainment in a bus or train but quietly, thoughtfully and calmly in your own home.

Most people automatically think a psychological problem is a difficult one to sort out. They don't start to work at a strategy and are quickly defeated before they really begin. Don't let this happen to you.

The resolution of psychological problems need not be more difficult than solving a physical one, unless you make it so.

You may feel that nothing can be done but you need to make a start somewhere. The following strategies are specifically targeted to get you moving.

1. Openly share anxieties and feelings with your friends, family and partner. If this doesn't work or is not possible, find someone, preferably a counsellor or a therapist.

2. Think about your problem, its root causes, why you are depressed and to what degree. Think also about any actions you have already taken to remedy it.

3. Talk the problem through with those involved: your husband; the family; the neighbours; colleagues at work (e.g. if you are being bullied or sexually harassed).

However depressed you are, to resolve it you will need to take a new and different viewpoint of yourself, build confidence and find a more secure sense of self.

If you have a self-image problem, you may have to eat more sensible and balanced meals, perhaps exercise regularly throughout the year. If you are worried about your health and have not already done so, it would be sensible to talk to your GP about it.

Look at the relationship with your partner, the quality of your sharing and caring. Look at the problems and how you can resolve them as a team effort.

If you are on your own, work out a strategy to go out more and to meet people. If you are shy or nervous, this can be attractive. Just be natural and yourself. Meet a man you find interesting and enjoy being with him.

Consider alternative therapy as an option. See the section at the end of the book.

Re-think the directions of your life. Take one step at a time rather than attempting several steps, in several directions, at the same time.

Consolidate each step you have taken before moving on. Make friends in new situations and only when you have made a commitment, move on to other new things.

There are a series of interactive sheets throughout the book, to help you solve your problems in a more practical, direct way.

RISE AND SHINE

Don't lie in bed until mid-morning or later. It will add to depressive feelings and you will feel less in control.

Get up at a reasonable time, stretch and salute the day. Just the action of getting up will make you feel better and you have already done something positive.

On waking, give your body a dry brush massage. Work upwards from the feet towards the heart. Brush downwards towards the heart from the neck, shoulders and upper back areas. This removes dead cells, stimulates the circulation and lymphatic drainage. Your skin will tingle and glow and you will feel more alive. Rub almond, olive, or peach kernel oil into any dry areas. Try mixing the oils and see which suits you best.

Use the energy of the morning to motivate yourself and to deal with the major chores of the day.

However busy you are, make time slots for yourself in the afternoon and evening, just to be relaxed and easy.

Pace yourself and maintain a relaxed, un-pressurised approach to the day. If you feel more energised in the evening use the drive for your own enjoyment. Only undertake a few of the chores you were too tired to face earlier in the day. At all times avoid depleting your energy reserves or overloading yourself.

Mobilise help from family or friends when this is a realistic possibility.

Don't complicate life, keep it simple and flowing.

ANYONE FOR TENNIS ?

Raise your fitness levels and you will feel less jaded. On waking, a ten minute work-out of back, tummy, hip and thigh stretch exercises is well worth the effort.

Walk, jog, swim or cycle for half-an-hour every day. Vary your routines and don't wrap-up excessively. Wear light, comfortable, loose, breathable clothing and shoes.

Exercise out of doors. The fresh air will help distance you from stress. As you merge with nature make a positive effort not to talk or think about your problems.

If you are obliged to exercise indoors open the windows and let a current of fresh air flow. Avoid a stuffy, airless environment at all times.

Strain and injury can be caused by prolonged, excessive exercising and using weights or fitness machines which are too heavy for you. A warm-up period and stretching are essential before beginning any form of exercise.

As you exercise blend with and become the movements and the breathing. Aim for a state of mind where your problems are no longer in charge or control you.

Avoid backing yourself into a psychological corner where it is impossible to perceive what changes you need to make. Narrow rigid thinking is often the cause.

Enjoy a brisk walk and fresh air each day, both are essential for health.

Keeping it simple will make life a lot easier.

FRESH JUICES WILL GIVE YOU A GLOW

Use fresh juices daily to give a boost to your vitality and to boost your sense of well-being. After two weeks your skin will start to glow, become more transparent and feel cleaner.

Drink a glass of vegetable juices twice a day. A cocktail of carrot, celery, apple, pear, kiwi, orange, peach or nectarine is beneficial. Whenever possible buy organic (non-sprayed) vegetables and fruit. Add fresh cranberries if you have a tendency to bladder problems. Use beetroot, carrot and apple for long-term problems.

Start to care for your body more but also put positive thoughts into your mind. Look for the insights and understanding which will allow a breakthrough in your thinking to occur and make change a reality. You will need to make the time and find a quiet, un-pressurised place for this to occur.

Try not to fragment your thoughts and feelings as you do this.

Look at the choice of modern juicers (preferably stainless steel) and buy one today. Use it daily.

Simplify, Simplify, Simplify, is the key to making fundamental changes in your thought processes and actions. Avoid intellectual traps or slick solutions which will not last. Keep your thinking very basic and focused. You can do it.

DON'T EAT ON THE HOOF

Eat some raw foods daily. A lunchtime large, mixed salad is ideal. Fruit and lightly steamed vegetables are also good for you. Reduce your intake of oven-ready, pre- cooked, frozen or convenience foods.

Eat quietly and slowly, preferably sitting down. Give yourself time to look, taste and enjoy. Avoid thinking or talking about your problems at meal times. Rushed, poorly digested meals are bad for your health and create gastric problems, a distraction from the more important psychological changes you need to make.

Don't try to do so much. Whenever possible aim to do less. Just be yourself and get outside your problems so that you can see them from a different angle and perspective. Spend time finding different ways and a different approach to achieve this.

Value and appreciate yourself as a unique person and ban all self-criticism.

Put yourself first rather than last and keep to it.

Feeling guilty or blaming yourself is negative and drains energy. It is usually a recurrent state of mind to confuse you and avoid change. Don't be taken in by it.

Develop attitudes which will take you forwards. Avoid despair or recurrent hopeless feelings taking over.
Become more positive and forward-looking in everything you do.

Simple and easy is the key.

GOODBYE MR CHIPS

Eat fatty, fried foods in strict moderation. If you have a weight problem they are best avoided until this has been resolved. Some unsaturated fats are good for you, especially cold-pressed olive oil.

To prevent weight gain and to stay fit and healthy, regular exercise is important, but keep it reasonable and not obsessional. On average exercise three times weekly for 30 minutes, provided you enjoy it and it is not excessive or damaging. Make the time for some exercise but give as much priority to changing your attitudes and moving forwards with your life.

Eat sensible balanced meals and don't diet when you are breast-feeding or have young children - it will add to exhaustion and stress. Bottled or filtered water is better for you than drinking endless cups of tea or coffee.

Lose those few extra pounds at a later date but control further weight gain by avoiding snacks and nibbles: especially crisps, chips, nuts, or salty savoury items.

Avoid a dietary regime which creates pressures or is likely to end in failure. Aim for a different approach and a new life style which is attainable and enjoyable.

Eating unhealthy foods is the same as taking in negative ideas which devalue you. Make changes in your eating habits but changing your self-attitude is even more important.

A simple, honest statement of your needs and priorities is always very helpful.

CUT THE SUGAR

Comfort eating when you feel tired or frustrated will lead to weight gain. If you crave sweet things eat a healthy orange or apple and avoid ice cream, cakes or biscuits and second helpings. Keep bread (wholemeal) intake to one slice with each meal. Potatoes are fine, steamed or baked. Keep your chocolate intake to sensible levels and only eat when you are hungry. Your teeth will also improve as an extra bonus.

A craving for sweet things is frequently a substitute for frustrated emotional needs. Look again at your relationship and ensure there is not a problem of communication, caring or sharing, which you are denying and not talking through.

Keep your weight at target levels for your height and age. Combine a regular exercise programme with sensible balanced eating habits, without dieting, which you can enjoy and sustain. Make healthy eating a part of your overall strategy for life.

Avoid becoming 'faddy' about food and dieting or your weight. A compulsion to devour everything in the fridge suggests you look again at any underlying frustration.

Make your meals enjoyable and sensible. Take smaller portions and eat lots of salad and fruit.

Encourage your taste buds to get to know simple, plain, tastes again and wean them off sugary items. They will soon lose the habit but do persist.

CANCEL THE PUFFER TRAIN

Smoking is an unhealthy, highly addictive habit which is best avoided. Don't just aim to cut down, it doesn't work. Break the habit completely and consider using nicotine patches as an aid to stopping.

If you are smoking because of tension, or lack of confidence, find a better way to boost your self-esteem. Work out your personal strategy for doing this before you stop. In this way there is less chance of failure.

Distrust any statement you make which says you enjoy smoking and don't want to give it up.

Throw away any store of surplus cigarettes or tobacco. Break the habit completely and persuade your partner to stop also. Avoid other addictive habits at this time, especially alcohol. It will tend to weaken your resolve.

Clarify any particular time of the day when you are most under pressure and take simple remedial steps e.g. meditation, relaxation, yoga, to reduce your stress levels.

Aim to become more of an individual and a person in your own right. Mix with non-smokers rather than smokers and keep informed about items such as salt, sugar, coffee, which may undermine your well-being or threaten the health of a future pregnancy or your family.

Simply stand by your determination, however strong the urge to go back to it. Work through the steps of stopping before you give up. It's not that difficult and it will boost your confidence and health.

RELAXEZ-VOUS

Relaxation is of enormous value and will help release drive and energy, reducing tension and stress levels with a positive effect on your vital reserves and ability to move forwards.

Relaxation and meditation, are some of the best ways to reduce stress and improve your overall health. Yoga, massage, reflexology, a creative hobby, are other ways.

Relax throughout the day and not just at certain times. As you do so, distance yourself from your problems. This will help you to stay relaxed at times of high demand or pressure e.g. when you are busy or driving.

Join a relaxation class in your area. You might also want to consider:- transcendental meditation, aromatherapy, health and fitness, or a mum's support group. The group experience is usually helpful and you will meet other mums, learning how they cope with stress and feelings similar to your own.

Find out about groups in your area and join one, or better still, start one yourself.

If you haven't the time to join a group, flop loosely on the carpet, your back to the floor and with legs and arms outstretched. Visualise yourself flowing and floating, warm, buoyant and at peace, as if lying on a cloud. Do this daily for ten minutes and take the phone off.

Simply aim to lose yourself totally during the process of relaxing.

THE INTERACTIVE SHEETS

The interactive sheets are your way of personalising the book and making it more real and relevant to your own particular symptoms and problem. They involve you more directly with what has been written, give you feedback and allow you to monitor your progress and change. In this way they help make the book more linked to you as an individual and your individual viewpoints and needs. It also allows you to take more charge of the themes of the book and to relate them directly to your own problem areas.

Adding your own input and ideas creates a more direct, personal experience which will help you respond to the ideas and stimulation of the book.

If you are feeling depressed and want to benefit from the book, fill in the sheets as directed as you go through the book. Each is linked to a different stage and depth of the book and is targeted to measure how much you have been able to make contact with different depths of feelings within yourself and how these relate to your depression. They will also give you a measure of the insights and changes you have made.

Give yourself a day to think quietly about each sheet and only then write down in detail your main feelings and areas of concern. In this way you can benefit from reading the book and also monitor the changes you have been able to make. There are six interactive sheets for mums and two for partners. When you are recording your personal details take your time, keep your ideas simple and don't rush.

17

INTERACTIVE SHEET 1 THE PROBLEM

date

**Write down your main symptoms of the 'blues'.
List them in order of importance.
Keep them brief, direct and to the point.
Make it simple and uncomplicated.**

1.

2.

3.

4.

Keep the sheets, simple, accurate and relevant.

DOCTOR, DOCTOR

Depression does not always have a psychological cause. It may be associated with a variety of physical conditions e.g. an infection, a low-functioning thyroid condition, toxic factors within the office environment, atmospheric pollution, exhaustion and burn-out following a prolonged period of deadlines, pressure and stress.

Intolerance to self-prescribed drugs bought over the counter at a chemist or supermarket may sometimes cause problems, or they may interact with a prescribed drug, alcohol, or a particular type of food, causing low mood symptoms.

Depression is common following childbirth or any illness which 'knocks the stuffing out of you' (causing a depleted state of vital reserves) e.g. after glandular fever, influenza, shingles. It can also occur after a severe illness or operation which exhausts you or requires a period of convalescence.

If in doubt ask for a full health check. You may be anaemic, have a hormonal imbalance or dietary allergic problem (e.g. to wheat). A simple iron tonic may be all you need to feel fit again.

Give yourself time, it may take several months for your reserves to fully recover when depleted. Always consider a simple, natural approach to health unless there is a specific condition which requires a specific treatment.

I'M ALRIGHT, IT'S THE BABY

If you are worried about your own or the baby's health, see your health visitor. Avoid allowing problems to accumulate which later get on top of you.

Many mums do not allow their own needs to be fully admitted and put the children and family first. Recurrent concerns about a minor condition of the baby can be an indirect and a psychological way of gaining help and attention, expressing a mum's fears about her own health and needs. Make sure you express those needs directly and openly.

Don't allow stress and anxiety levels to build up and develop a power base where they can undermine confidence and cause symptoms.

Aim for a direct and complete expression of all your emotions, keeping them clear, simple and flowing.

Clarify and keep separate your own needs and personality from those of the baby and your partner.

Everyone has feelings, they are part of being human and they should not be suppressed or seen as something to hide or feel ashamed of. Try not to deny any of your emotions.

Look to see if there are any areas where you are displacing feelings into other situations or people. Take steps to rectify this before it causes confusion or harm.

Simplify your approach to life, needs and emotions.

FINDING SOLUTIONS

Many of the problems we create are based on fear of what might happen if we challenge established norms and authority. The majority of these anxieties are not based on reality and their main function is to create a situation of hesitation, doubt and fear. As a result, nothing is done and change is avoided.

If you become intimidated or passive this tends to lock you into a position where movement, change and challenge are much more difficult to achieve. Don't allow problems or imaginative fears to build-up and swamp you. If you are in any way worried about your own physical or psychological health, just telephone your doctor or the Well Woman Clinic.

Look closely at any tendency to avoid or delay taking decisions or making a significant change in your life. Clarify how long this has been happening and evolve a strategy to change and modify it. Note if avoidance and finding excuses only happens at times of stress and 'major' events or if there is a tendency for this to occur at other times.

Talk about any underlying loss of confidence but also about doing things differently, daring to challenge and experiment and to open up with new suggestions and new ideas. Find ways to implement this part of you and to make it a living reality.

Visualise yourself into a position of confidence and change. Allow it to happen. Keep it simple.

I'M LATE, I'M LATE

Avoid being fussed by housework. At the same time don't let a mountain of washing, ironing or dishes accumulate. Find an alternative to becoming either a slave to household chores or a 'slut'.

Free yourself from endless chores. They will drag you down and put a stop to the more healthy creative aspects of your individuality.

Tidy up adequately but no more than this. Keep some free time for yourself and use it enjoyably. Use careful planning and preparation to set yourself boundaries and build in time for your own needs to relax and to have a quiet space.

Avoid losing your identity under an avalanche of jobs around the house or washing-up.

Obsessional neatness, like obsessional thinking, ties you down and it is more about imposing controls than change and growth or achieving your potential.

Stop the chores treadmill while you still have time and use the energy to enjoy fun things and to expand your ideas and develop your originality. Remain on top of the housework chores rather than allowing them to accumulate and to overwhelm you.

There is no need ever to feel guilty or to deny that you get tired and have needs and priorities.

Be radical and keep it simple and to the point.

PLAYING SUPERMUM

Running a home, the family, having children is tiring and it takes a lot out of you. Pace yourself, plan more and reduce unnecessary household chores.

A short, ten minutes sleep in the afternoon is nearly always beneficial. So go for it.

Avoid being over-ambitious, doing too much or exhausting yourself. Don't try to be omnipotent by driving yourself to extremes.

Many mums have a tendency to push themselves to the limit. They inevitably become exhausted and depleted, then feel a failure because they need to rest but won't allow themselves to do so. This is because it is seen as weakness and 'giving in'.

There is little point in pushing yourself to the limit if you are already tired and only just coping with the basics you have to get through.

Supermums are a danger to themselves because they deny their own basic needs. Make sure your family knows that you do your best but like all members of the family team, you need time and space for your own feelings, interests and projects.

Admit when you feel tired and rest. Avoid the trap of playing Supermum. It is not worth the risk. Keep it plain and simple.

THIS PLACE FEELS LIKE A PRISON

A strict, repressive upbringing may have meant that the expression of your individuality and needs was not fully allowed.

As a child you may have already erected an emotional wall, making you 'up tight' or depressed. The family home can come to reflect those inner feelings and become like a prison.

Mums easily become depressed because of the demands of the children, especially a new baby, often becoming debilitated. Lack of energy inevitably means lack of confidence, irritability and sometimes thoughts of violence.

If you have any of these feelings, discuss them with your partner and avoid withdrawal. You may need a break if you are over tired. Often you are the only person who can really assess how tired and jaded you really are.

Look again at your dreams and the language you use when discussing your home. This may give some clues about the origin of those depressive feelings. Make time to explore and expand these feelings and the more repressed or inhibited aspects of your personality.

Don't keep yourself or your feelings under wraps. All mums feel depressed at times and it is normal to feel this way and not something to be ashamed of. The real priority is releasing an inner trapped you. Stay direct and simple (meaning stay yourself), while the changes are happening. Enjoy.

FLY ME TO THE MOON

However much you enjoy your home everyone needs a break at times, new surroundings and contacts. This creates a natural pause and allows you to re-charge your batteries with a break from routine.

If getting away from the home environment is a priority and will make you feel better, then don't hesitate. Take a break and don't feel guilty about it. Visit your local art gallery, museum, cinema, park or have lunch with a friend. Get away for a weekend visiting friends or family, perhaps a health farm.

Aim for a complete change of people and scenery. Try to do this on a regular basis, at least once a month.

Build variety and change into your daily life. Enjoy activities with your children and as a family but also with your partner and sometimes alone or with friends.

Retain your interests, at all times keeping an open alert mind. Make all aspects of your life favourable to new ideas, to explore, experiment and develop. Ensure you create the time and physical space (at least a table and chair) for this to occur. Keep this as your private place for ideas and projects and to stimulate your mind.

Keep your day simple, pleasurable and active, the ideas flowing. Make simple models of your projects and try to develop them. Always discuss them with your children as this will encourage them to do likewise. They may even come up with some new ideas which will link with your own.

BACK TO BASICS

Clarify the main reasons why and when problems occur and work out ways to anticipate and defuse them. Sort out any neglected emotional areas, often involving the quality and priority of your communication and sharing with your partner, or the family. Think them through again and put them into a new perspective which allows you to make changes and to move on in the present and the future.

If there is a specific area which is worrying you, try to see how it originated and why it has come up at this time, also what other aspects of your life it is affecting. Discuss the problems with your partner and consider any ideas he may have.

Look clearly at other periods in your life when you also found it hard to resolve a difficulty. Look clearly at the reasons then and how much you have matured and moved on in confidence and experience since that time.

A direct approach to problem solving will build experience and make you feel stronger and more sure of yourself.

Write down or say out loud the options and choices open to you. What are your priorities at this time?

Put these into action. Avoid delaying tactics and passivity. At all times keep it very simple and uncomplicated. Just let it go and flow with it.

IF I WERE A RICH MAN

Don't allow money matters and making ends meet to dominate your whole thinking, or become a source of panic with fears of everything collapsing around you.

Treat financial problems in a practical way and don't allow them to become symbols of success or failure, or a reason to change your fundamental beliefs. If you have a debt problem and are under pressure, re-schedule the payments and as far as is practical, aim to clear it within a period of months.

Try not to borrow and only spend what you can afford. You will probably find you can get by spending less than you had previously thought. Addictive spending is a common problem which quickly builds up. It is often related to underlying frustration or depression and the need for short-term satisfactions and reassurance. Lack of confidence and a compulsive need to do something or take some action is a common cause.

If you begin to value and accept yourself more you will also find that problems become less threatening and can be more easily resolved. Look again at any emotional issues which in the past have contributed to the problem and make changes and adjustments to prevent this happening again in the future.

Share the problems and work out the solutions together. If necessary get professional help and advice - from Social Services, your bank manager or the Citizens Advice Bureau.

Discuss financial matters in a simple, sensible way.

A VERY SPECIAL MUM

It is a crowning achievement to be a mum. You are lucky to be one and very special. Appreciate what you have done and be kind to yourself. Be proud of your contribution to humanity, the start you have given to a human life. Enjoy it, even if at times it can be tiring and demanding.

See your children as the fruit of your femininity and that you have given the gift of life and opportunity. Learn to enjoy and value yourself more and don't make it conditional on age, appearance, background, or experience.

If you are alienated from your child (or children) make every attempt to contact them and be prepared to welcome them when you see them again.

If a child has died and you are feeling depressed, think of the positive things which occurred and that not every seed can develop into a mature plant. Accept life with its gains and losses as a part of the whole, the inevitable shape of things. Try not to feel resentful towards others you feel are more fortunate, or to feel guilty.

Show just how much you value yourself by arranging a luxury day out. Pamper yourself and enjoy being you. Don't only make this a one-off but aim to do it on a regular basis. It should emphasise how much you matter and be an appreciation of your intrinsic needs. You should come back refreshed and re-invigorated.

Allow yourself to move forwards and on.

INTERACTIVE SHEET 2 THE REASONS
date

Write down what you consider to be the main contributing reasons for the present difficulties. Include both recent and past events and list them in order of their relevance to your becoming depressed.

1.

2.

3.

4.

Keep your comments spontaneous, linked to your own feelings and experience but especially keep them simple.

NO MUM IS AN ISLAND

Avoid losing your identity and skills within the demands and routines of family life. Maintain your identity as you extend your artistic, intellectual and social contacts.

Develop new interests and ideas and make time for them to be shared and expressed. Spend part of every day exploring something new, creative and experimental.

Aim for full involvement with your family and those close to you but not swamped or swallowed up by them. In this way, you can continue to grow, expand and develop as an individual as well as a family unit.

Avoid becoming isolated because of language or cultural problems or the needs of a young family. Retain links with your traditions and past roots as well as freeing the impetus to move forward in the present and the future. Shun any tendency to be inward looking or to withdraw by a determination to expand, move forward and on.

Find a place within yourself where you feel strong, secure and at peace. Experience this strength and allow it to grow and expand. Spend quiet time with an inner you and get to know its strengths and the individuality it expresses. Feed it with cultural and artistic links and expand into confidence, achievement, reality and happiness.

Be bold, daring and imaginative. Allow yourself to move forwards as a person. Don't let fear or lack of confidence hold you back. Use these as simple tools to progress with and as a positive advantage rather than a brake or negative factor.

WEARING BLINKERS

Focus on those aspects where you feel most confident but also look at any areas where you have difficulties or blockage. Narrow, rigid attitudes can limit your outgoing, explorative self. Nourish all elements of your being, the physical as well as psychological sides of yourself and those around you.

Create an environment of peace, where there are no barriers or no-go areas, so that each member of the family can explore and develop. Feel free to question, agree or disagree with different points of view, to express ideas, feelings and emotions at all levels. Also create the resources for growth within yourself and expand an inner environment where trust, affection, communication, personal belief and faith can grow and flourish.

Clarify how your emerging ideas and perceptions are modified and moulded by the way you perceive and think and the influences of others, including the media. Focus on how this erodes creative ideas, drives and health. Work out a strategy to prevent this happening.

Create a personal time-table which can be modified, one which allows you to continue to develop and reach your personal targets and potential without having to compromise on the needs of your children or the family in any way. Make it something they can participate in without formal or rigid limits. Let this emerge from you as a vitality, an inner presence which you radiate and which can nourish and encourage those around you.

Aim for simplicity in all things.

EVERY ILLNESS IS A JOURNEY

The resolution of depression is a journey of discovery which can throw light on a process which for years has kept you marginalised and from fully realising your inner identity and self.

Life is essentially about change, growth, movement, energy conservation and its release. New ideas, thoughts, understanding, perceptions and evolving aims are inherent within you and vital to a healthy existence. Experience yourself as a kaleidoscope of rich images, perceptions and feelings of many tones and colours. This will give you a glimpse into your inner world and its varied and meaningful totality.

See your present state of mind as a pivotal point on a journey of change, a crisis which centres around the process of movement and renewal. For some it is their first real expression of individuality, a first rebellion and a first authentic expression of self.

The ability to experience and express a sense of self is the key to psychological health. For many it is the dawn of a new beginning, a new shape and renewed hope. A break with the past and past thinking leads to new skills and new perceptions developing, the ability to be free from a previously narrow vision of the world which led to frustration, unhappiness and a sense of failure.

Open up your mind to a new sequence of thoughts and awareness. Find ways to express the many different aspects of your make-up and being, to resolve this problem and get well. At the same time, retain a sense of simplicity in all things.

MY ILLNESS, MY CURE

The admission of difficulties and learning how to turn around a depressive problem has an enormous positive value for growth and change. The 'blues' should not just be seen as something negative or an illness. A breakdown often heralds a 'break away' and a 'break through', the first steps back to becoming more confident and integrated. Understand how this applies to you and communicate it to yourself and others.

Every illness is a pause, a crisis and a challenge but above all, it is a powerful potential for expansion, moving forward and renewal. The experience of illness is not always an easy one. For many it is the first significant expression of need and self and a cry for help. The recognition that previous blinkered or rigid attitudes led nowhere or produced an isolated, unhappy, frustrated life can be a very rewarding experience.

A sense of freedom comes from the ability to move forwards again, into a stronger and more authentic way of seeing and being.

To avoid a return to old attitudes and perceptions you will have to be vigilant. However the very positive experience of working through a crisis brings new strengths, a new learning process and new insights to prevent a recurrence, the door is opened and the lock turned.

Think positively. Even in the depths of despair don't lose hope. However turbulent the winds of depression or doubt, maintain confidence and direction. Stay on course, stay you and stay simple.

LOOK FOR THE POSITIVE

Keep a balance in all things including your optimism, faith and belief in yourself. Maintain contact with a positive self. This will allow you to deal with powerful emotions such as rage, jealousy, envy or rebellious feeling which might otherwise overwhelm you.

See the 'blues' as related to a sense of loss and isolation from your essential self. The lack of contact undermines happiness and confidence, causing a fudged sense of self-identity and being. Alienation can lead to confusion, despair, loss of the drive to move forwards as well as loss of contact with yourself.

When your sense of self feels weak or taken over, you more easily feel dragged down by the weight of your problems and unable to rise above them. Separate yourself from the problems of the moment and maintain contact with others and a more healthy balanced part of you.

Even in a severely depressed situation mobilise your adult positive self so that you are not dominated by negative feelings. These are often infantile in origin and re-create well-worn patterns with childish feelings of defeat, anger and despair. Work with those feelings rather than against them and see them as a part of you which needs reassurance and support. This will give you a more positive approach, more confidence, better control and a sense of working towards change. You may have to live with these feelings for some time but they will eventually mature and become less threatening.

Stay simple and centred and balanced in all things.

THREE LETTER WORD

If you had a rigid upbringing where sex was regarded as a dirty word, this may have caused hang-ups and difficulties in the past. Make sure you share any problems in this area with your partner and don't hide away your needs, sexual urges, phantasies or feelings.

If there is a sexual problem clarify where the problem lies and discuss it openly. Don't force yourself into a difficult or blocked situation. Allow all your feelings to flow and to be expressed. Many sexual problems are infantile in origin and based on omnipotent phantasies which create a distorted model of the world and others. Try to see where and how they act and the bias they bring, at the same time continuing to express yourself as you are and feel.

Look again at your childhood or teenage experiences and see if there are any no-go areas you have not accepted or forgiven. Avoid being blocked by an unhappy past and move into a fuller expression of yourself in the present. Clinging to the past from fear or a 'bad' experience is often based on flight from being you in the now and blocks your ability to renew yourself at all levels of expression and caring.

If anger was locked away at the time of a childhood hurt or trauma and was not talked about or became linked to shame and guilt, it may still be feared. This can create a block to health, closeness, trust, caring and loving.

A simple, uncomplicated expression of your feelings and needs is always best.

TRUST IS KEY TO HEALTH

Many problems of depression in mums of all ages, are related to a disturbed relationship with their partner. Lack of open communication, the amount of time spent together, commitment, sharing, openness, talking and understanding are some of the key factors. These are the building blocks of a healthy unit which can work through and discuss problems jointly and either solve them or work towards a better approach and outcome. Each partner brings the strengths, understanding and different skills to focus upon a difficulty. This also enhances your skills of sharing and working together in other areas, including pleasure, enjoyment and sex.

Be honest with yourself about the relationship with your partner and quite certain there is not a problem of closeness, sharing, or communication which is being denied. Ensure you are open with each other, especially about any doubts or fears, concerning the quality of the caring which exists and your ability to move together as a unit, a partnership and a couple.

Make today a target day to examine and think about how clearly and directly you express yourself. This will not only help in the present but also towards repairing an unsatisfactory or painful past. You can't change the past, only the way you feel about it but you can make changes in the present.

You may not be able to change the past but you can change your feelings, perceptions and attitudes to it, which is fundamentally about changing you as a person. Once you understand this it will simplify many other areas in your life.

SHED THOSE TEARS

Tears are a normal and healthy expressions of emotion for men as well as women. They reflect your sensitivity and your human qualities.

Don't hide away tears or indeed any aspect of yourself including rage, irritability or frustration. Have a good cry and let go without feeling shame or guilt. At the same time aim to understand your tears and what they are expressing and the reasons for them. Avoid crying in private.

Free any trapped and unexpressed aspects of yourself - fears, feelings, needs, ideas, hopes, dreams, phantasies - and talk about them with your partner, friends and family. Make sure you have a clear understanding what these are and ask yourself whether they are aspects of yourself you find acceptable or if you feel guilty and ashamed of them.

Tears express adult hurts, rage and disappointment as well as infantile needs, fears and frustration. Whatever their origin they need to have life and to be expressed. If you wish their maturity and appropriateness can be discussed at a later time but let them out now.

If you feel upset simply share it and show it. Clarify any links with an unsatisfactory past or upbringing when it feels right and relevant.
Give priority at all times to the expression of how you feel and who you are. Don't hide away or attack yourself.

LET ME OUT

Don't lock feelings away like a genie in a bottle. Any denial of emotions is a denial of yourself and can lead to panic or an undermining of confidence.

As soon as you lock feelings away you have also locked away and isolated parts of yourself. Because they no longer have a check or balance on reality those isolated feelings can become an issue in themselves, a pocket of blocked emotional energy and drive which develops its own particular brand of logic and assumptions about others, which is not always based on reality. As a result they can easily become excessive and frightening and feel out of control, leading to tension and sometimes illness.

Open every line of communication with your partner but don't alienate him by their strength or demanding intensity.

If your major needs are for support, a listening ear and for your partner to be there, help him understand this. Be ready also to listen to and support his needs and fears as well as your own.

Clarify that you want to share your feelings and you are not seeking an intellectual analysis of the problems, or asking him to become another Sigmund Freud or the prophet Solomon.

Make sure he understands your needs are: to be listened to, to talk and share feelings, to be accepted as you are. Avoid pressurising and keep it simple.

COAT OF MANY COLOURS

Maintain contact with others and avoid withdrawing, or allowing phantasies to take over or dominate your mind and rational thinking. You need to be aware of both and at the same time to keep a balance.

Broaden the base of your relationships by developing new creative interests and activities. Keep these simple and direct. You are aiming at expressing and sharing feelings, getting closer to others, giving out more of yourself, being able to care and to show it. This is not a difficult or complicated process, it is being and expressing your natural self.

See your feelings as resembling wave patterns with peaks and troughs, swings and eddies, pulling you to one side or the other, lateral currents, funnels of energy, froth and foam, periods of turmoil and all the time variations in their overall pattern and intensity.

Let yourself flow like a river of feelings and ideas towards a greater sense of confidence and awareness, individuality, peace and wholeness. Your ultimate goal is a realisation of your own uniqueness in all its different colours, shapes and forms.

Talk, share, give and confide for greater self-expression and self-realisation. Be as open and spontaneous as possible. Spend more time listening rather than talking. Try to avoid superficial chatting in order to placate or keep the peace, cover-up the whole problem area, or create barriers rather than building trust, sharing and closeness. It simply is not worth it.

41

INTERACTIVE SHEET 3 THE ACTIONS
date

Write down any actions you are taking in order to make changes and to remedy your 'blues' situation. List them in order of importance.

1.

2.

3.

4.

Keep it brief, to the point, basic and simple.

DON'T LIVE IN A CLOSET

If you feel down about a particular issue clarify the causes and what needs to be done. Make each step an easy, natural progression and avoid turning it into a threat, terror, or nightmare.

Self-criticism, a fruitless search for perfection and fear of failure, are some of the most common attitudes used to delay making changes. They can totally defeat your ability to resolve problems, clarify ideas or reach a more enlightened understanding of yourself. Depression is often caused by a persistent denial of what needs to be done and the understanding, perceptions and ideas which are basic to health.

Your thought processes quite naturally flow and link up with feelings and emotions to create new shapes, new concepts and a new evolving you. If this basic process becomes blocked or aspects of you become side-lined, denied, or suppressed it can feel quite devastating, rather like a loss of your identity, or the death of you as a functioning person and likely to lead to depression.

This kind of blockage is mainly directed at blocking change but it keeps you like a cabbage and creates feelings of defeat and despair. Try to avoid this happening and give every side of your being the chance to emerge, to have its say and a life.

Stop slamming the door on change. Be prepared to change any rigid defeatist attitudes. Break the inner log-jam, open the lock gates, start to flow and to live again. Don't make it complicated, and keep it very simple and natural.

ROUTINES WHICH KEEP YOU CAPTIVE

It may sometimes be impossible to get away totally from the demands and pressures of a young family. If routines are getting on top of you, at least take a break psychologically, distancing yourself from the immediate problems and chores.

If you are feeling in a rut it is often because you have stopped thinking laterally and creatively and are only functioning in a repetitive, circular way of thinking. This locks you into a fixed way of being and responding, undermining your ability to be flexible and to make shifts and changes.

Think yourself into a more positive attitude. Examples might be: your last good holiday, enjoyable sex, that special meal you had together, one you plan to make.

Vary your routines and change your patterns. Each day practice some form of relaxation or meditation. Make more time to enjoy, read, write, make and do. Most of all change your mood by contacting a more inner resilient, positive you and ensure it has a viable outlet of expression.

Avoid the conventional and the predictable. Think differently. Evolve a strategy to make changes in your relationships and your life. Don't let routines take over.

Free yourself totally from worry for one glorious day. Do the same for the next day and the next. Continue to move on and to develop as you do so. It's as simple as that.

GUILTY

Tease out any guilt feelings and bring them into the light of day. Find out (preferably with your partner) where they originated and if the feelings are appropriate or make any sense at all. If you feel guilty about insensitive behaviour make changes in the future but ensure you are not attacking yourself for being direct, honest and blunt about what you feel is right.

If your guilt feelings are excessive or harsh you are probably making too severe judgements about yourself. This is probably happening in other areas too as a punishing, hard-line conscience tries to dominate and control you. It is probably also directed to other members of the family who step over the line or express new, challenging thoughts and ideas.

Ensure you are not identifying with the patterns of another member of the family e.g. a parent, becoming like them and perpetuating an old mythology which preserves the past and is frightened of moving on.

The unrealistic demands of a punishing conscience (your inner standards officer) may refuse to allow you any freedom. This causes irritability and frequent problems with others because it does not tolerate anyone else making a mistake either. Clarify how this limits you.

Locate within yourself, at least one key reason for changing and wanting to resolve your present problems.

Don't allow a punishing conscience to spoil your life by blocking all the enjoyment and fun of your relationships and creative drives.

THE S-WORD

Admit you are sorry when you are in the wrong but don't allow guilt or resentment to fester. Keep any guilt feelings in balance and on a short lead. Be vigilant when they come up, ensuring they are appropriate and make good sense. They may try to liaise with other perfectionist traits you have or search for unattainable ideals rather than a dynamic, attainable, flexible reality.

Apologise in order to move on but make sure you do discuss feelings which need to come up and you are not retreating to a safe area which is not going anywhere.

Apologise quickly and sincerely and avoid being dominated by pride. Others will soon let you know if it is uncalled for. The airing of feelings will help clear the air and is therapeutic. At the same time beware of masochism, feelings of self-punishment or inappropriate guilt. These can trap you into passivism and inactivity.

Avoid old familiar feelings of guilt which have no relevance in the present e.g. those which link back to childhood and the past and are not part of the thrust forwards of a healthy, balanced, dynamic you.

The s-word is also the sex or sin word and these are often linked to guilt feelings, creating confusion and uncertainty, blocking momentum and the dynamic new.

We all make mistakes. Apologise if you really feel it. But remember - you are not a saint and even if you idealise him - neither is your partner.

IF YOU DON'T ENJOY IT, SAY SO

Some mums don't always feel like full (vaginal) sex for some time after the birth. There are many reasons for this including pain, hormonal factors, psychological worries, fear of conceiving and tiredness. Lack of confidence is a common factor or it is sometimes linked to lack of privacy, especially when a young baby or a member of the family is sleeping in a nearby room.

If you are not enjoying sex say so and don't feel you have to pretend. Avoid putting up with anything you can't enjoy or fully participate in.

Don't make direct physical, sexual love your sole priority and outcome of your intimacy. Try enjoying new and different pleasures e.g. lying close, reading to each other, listening to quiet music together. At times in order to stimulate the phantasies, you may want to share an erotic video or magazine; or just have an early night and wake early.

Try to see sexuality within a much wider context linked to trust, bonding and closeness, the quality of your openness, communication and sharing. The confidence you were able to develop as a child is also relevant and parental attitudes to sexual exploration and games has an important input on your present day attitudes.

Discuss this with your partner and be creative, developing other less direct sexual activities: quiet holding, massage, mutual intimate caresses, stroking, a vibrator, lying close in a relaxed way. Switch the TV off. You can try oysters, but make sure they are in season. You make the choices.

LOVE IS A MANY-SIDED THING

You are unlikely to feel exactly the same kind of idealised love and enchantment towards your partner as when you first met - because no one does.

At times you are likely to feel hostile, irritable and ambivalent. These feelings are common to everyone and may need to come to the surface and be expressed. Emotions and needs change and evolve constantly. Be prepared for this and expect it to happen.

The arrival of a new baby may make your partner feel threatened, needing reassurance that he matters. If he feels insecure or sees the new baby as a rival for your affections, he may also exhibit baby-like (regression) behaviour in order to gain attention. Some examples are developing similar symptoms to the baby e.g. indigestion, heartburn or burping. He may develop a new tendency to suck more, on pencils or a pipe, or perhaps become more childish, emotional and fretful, taking up your time and attention.

A period of hurt, pain or disappointment may lead to greater closeness and understanding. A deeper bonding can occur as you get through it together.

Reassure your partner (and if necessary the children). Explain that they matter as before and that the arrival of a new baby is an extension and part of them and not a threat to your love or caring for them. Be prepared to give your partner and also the children extra time in order to reassure them. Make sure your own physical and emotional needs are also well catered for and not neglected.

STAND BY YOUR MAN

Listen, stay close and give him support, understanding and time. Remember he is just as vulnerable as you are so don't over-pressurise him. Everyone needs their own time and space to reflect and for quiet thinking.

Communication increases security and confidence but don't lose your opinion and identity. Stay close but not sucked-in or swallowed-up by his viewpoints or anxieties.

Be prepared to express yourself clearly and assertively; if necessary to argue and to disagree. If you feel he is wrong, too narrow in his thinking, going over the top in his reactions, tell him and help him to see things from a different angle without imposing on him. It sounds difficult but it isn't, provided you keep your communications simple, direct and to the point.

Stand by yourself too, your integrity as a person, your ability to repair and care for yourself. Show your thoughts and ideas but especially show your feelings and reactions. Allow him to bounce off you into a new and healthier position of understanding and perception.

Ask yourself: what is our vision for the future, our philosophy, beliefs, ambition and direction? Also ask: what is the point of our relationship and why and where are we going?

Stand by him but don't become him. Help him to find himself, his directions, priorities and needs. Don't hold back on the expression of your caring. Simply be you, the person you are and aspire to be.

NOTHING IS FOREVER

Don't automatically feel guilty or blame yourself if your relationship is no longer progressing and going forward with shared aims and directions. Try to talk through the main areas of the problem, giving time and priority to discussion and repair.

If you are unable to work together as a couple and feel blocked and unfulfilled, it may be better to have a period of separation. Where there is a severe breakdown of communication and you no longer feel happy or at ease with your partner, then consider a temporary separation but always discuss this openly.

You should feel as free about moving out as when you first moved in together. Get professional advice and keep informed of your rights. Be prepared to act on them but try to get back together as soon as communications and difficulties improve or have been resolved.

If this does not lead to better sharing, openness and communication, the ability to work together as a unit and a team, then it may be better to consider divorce and finding someone you can love, be a friend to, work and feel fulfilled with.

Ambivalent feelings are natural and in us all. They are an important part of our broad spectrum of feelings as well as the drive towards change.

Don't stay in a bad relationship where you are devalued, abused, rejected, or unhappy. It simply is not worth it.

51

REPAIR JOB

Every relationship has its problems and from time to time becomes jaded and flat, usually because you are tired, it has been neglected and taken for granted or takes second place to the pressures of the family and the job. If you give it priority, more time and appreciation, start to do things together again as a team, there is a good chance it will form itself into a more caring unit and you will be able to move forward again.

To keep your relationship supple and healthy you will need to do some form of on-going work, especially at openness and sharing. This in itself is therapeutic and sets the tone for the future. The work should be done jointly and not just be the responsibility of one partner, so that he or she feels at fault and needs to make all the changes and adjustments for the success of the marriage. Any problem areas which you discuss should certainly fully involve both of you.

If you have a relationship problem spend more time with each other, talking it through and exploring the fundamental problems and the differences between you. Don't bury your head in the sand or destroy yourself for the sake of security or fear - you may damage yourself and the children. Only stay together if you really want to, still care and are able to grow together. Make allowances that no one is perfect and that others make the same mistakes and cause the same hurts as you.

Work in a simple, straightforward way at your relationship and improve the quality of communication between you. Always aim for greater openness, sharing, trust and caring.

BABY BLUES

Many mums feel 'down' after the birth because they are tired, in pain, the baby cries at night and a jaded 'reality' sets in of the commitment she has made.

A mum can easily become isolated and feel guilty because of ambivalent feelings towards her partner or the baby, sometimes both. The feelings are made worse because she is usually unprepared for them, or compares herself with other mums who she imagines to be in an idyllic state of well being and fulfilment. If she does not quite share the myth she can begin to feel a failure and different from other mums. She may imagine she is failing her partner and the baby.

Should you develop any of these feelings make sure you share them with your partner and family and avoid hiding any negative feelings about yourself or the baby. If you have a previous history of post-natal depression it may recur after another delivery, or never happen again. If you move into a new area with a new GP be quite sure he is fully aware of your past history.

During any future pregnancies avoid putting too much stress or pressure on yourself or becoming over-tired. Be on your guard for any early symptoms of anxiety, depression or compulsive ideas.

Before and during your next pregnancy 'spring clean' your mind. Discuss with your partner any unresolved areas of conflict, guilt, emotion from the past or anything that is worrying you from more recent times.

Simple prevention is always better than cure.

INTERACTIVE SHEET 4. THE CHANGES
date
Note any changes that have occurred in your symptoms since reading the book and starting to take more positive action. List where there has been most change. Also list those areas where there has been little or no change and the problem is static or worse.
Changes have occurred in:-.

1.

2.

3.

4.

No change, or a worsening has occurred in the following areas:-

1.

2.

3.

4.

Keep all comments simple, to the point and honest.

LAME DUCK

Maintain your network of friends and don't lose your personality or become isolated by marriage, the children or the family. It is better to avoid turning yourself into a 'cabbage' as this will reinforce your negative self-imagery and your doubts.

Explore a wide variety of interests, new ideas and new contacts, preferably now rather than in the future. Ensure that you have a balanced, healthy image of yourself. If you feel inferior, a 'freak' or failure, plan moves and initiatives in order to boost your confidence.

Give yourself time to change and evolve. You will find it much more difficult in a vacuum and in isolation so make plans to improve your social life and keep to them. Developing wider interests, voluntary work, helping others, will also help to build your self-esteem.

If you are on your own without a partner make time to go out and meet others. Join a fitness club, special interest group, a new sport, go dancing. Do something which will bring you more into contact with other people and make new friendships in all the age groups. Enjoy their company and be a friend to them.

Avoid struggling on in a relationship which holds no genuine interest or future for you. You will know this because: there are no areas of mutual interest, you feel unfulfilled or unhappy, sexual attraction is absent, humour is lacking and your areas of shared interest and enjoyment are minimal or non-existent. Take simple decisions where these are obvious and long overdue.

THE PAST IMPERFECT

We all make mistakes, wrong moves and at times cause pain and suffering to others. It is inevitable and part of learning and maturing, the human experience.

Make sure that you learn from your mistakes and can forgive others. Don't let the past weigh too heavily on you so that it becomes a burden which blocks you and prevents you from moving on in the now. If you are constantly retracing and resenting the past it is destructive because it prevents you learning from it and feeling gratitude, as well as anger, for what it taught you. Whatever the past reach out and move on with your life.

Make sure you stay resilient and look forward to new beginnings and living in the now, rather than staying trapped and a victim of the past. Acknowledge any areas of hurt and rejection which still cause you pain but try not to dwell on them.

Hanging on to old traumas and disappointments will damage your self-confidence and it won't put the clock back. If you want to move on it is important to allow the past, the hurts and the regrets to fall away. This can be an effective way of removing blocks and freeing yourself.

Soften those old spoilers - resentment, perfection and control. Develop new, different attitudes to what has happened in the past. Look forward to unfolding a new, more positive mature you. It's that simple.

BRIDGE OF HEALING

Make changes and concessions. Build bridges to heal old rifts and resentments within yourself. Talk through and modify defensive, rigid attitudes which trap and block you in your relationships with others or prevent a forward flow of ideas, movement and growth.

Take a closer look at any feelings of hurt, anger or revenge you hold. They are often linked to those you are particularly close to, especially your family, siblings, partner and sometimes your children. Ensure you are not holding on to old resentments which block you and keep you distant and alienated. Avoid becoming a power freak, or taking the moral high ground.

This is one of the most important tasks you will ever undertake. In an imperfect world, there are bound to be some misunderstandings, ambivalent feelings and mistakes made. Stay humorous, be direct and sharp.

Make allowances and be prepared to forget and forgive. If not you will be tied down by life's sticks and stones, the inevitable imperfections of yourself and others, rather than becoming freed from them.

Take a more lateral approach to solving your problem. See yourself in five years time and envisage the steps you need to make it a reality. Next see yourself as having already arrived there and look back at the steps which you have taken to make it a success and a reality. Focus on those steps and implement one of them now.

Allow a simple, new, more natural, relaxed and mature you to emerge. Enjoy.

GREAT EXPECTATIONS

Free yourself from parental expectations and family, social and peer group pressures. Achieve independence by making a definite statement of your directions and intentions and where you stand. Encourage the emergence of your interests but also a softer, more caring intuitive self to emerge.

Allow feelings of need, love and anger to flow.

Express yourself as you are and not as others want you to be or as they would like you to have been. Live in the present and the new, expressing a wide spectrum of thoughts and ideas. These relate to the direction you are travelling in now and how free you are to explore and to create.

Avoid living in the past. Resist conforming to other people's expectations of what you should be. It may be a comfort and a reassurance to them but it does not help you develop or find yourself.

Free yourself from any constraints which impinge upon you as an individual, your ability to make choices and to move forwards. Make sure this reflects you as you are.

Expect the best and achieve it by being positive in your thinking and clear about your goals. Visualise them clearly and think through the steps to get you there. Live in the present and not in the future or the past.

Be yourself, as you are and as you feel and experience yourself.

DOCTOR MUM

A young doctor mum had a four year old daughter with recurrent chest infections, diagnosed by her colleague as bronchiolitis (an infection of the small breathing channels of the lung). The child was prescribed repeat antibiotics by the colleague and had been admitted to hospital on several occasions for observation and a variety of tests. The recurrent illnesses caused the mum anxiety and she became increasingly depressed about the child's health. In desperation, she took the child to see a homoeopathic doctor who prescribed a remedy for the mother's stress and anxiety and nothing for the child. As the mother became more relaxed and less depressed the child's chest condition cleared up completely and the bronchiolitis did not recur.

Tension and stress in any mum has a powerful undermining effect upon the physical and psychological health of her child. It is important to stay alert to the possibility of the child or her partner identifying with her symptoms and becoming ill or underfunctioning.

A physical or psychological problem in a child may be the first indication that the mum is depressed and needs help. Children are very sensitive and quickly pick up the vibes of their mum, whether she is happy or sad, feeling well or ill. They can start to worry about her state of mind, happiness and state of health. If a child identifies with a mum's sadness, it may become disturbed and anxious or develop physical symptoms.

Simple talking and explanation will often prevent a child taking on the tensions of the family.

MIND GAMES

Even in a severely depressed state of mind try to retain an overall responsibility for your feelings. Don't delegate total responsibility of your mind, ideals, goals and individuality to others.

Participate in the exploration of your problem but not in its manipulation or any process which damages your confidence and identity, or belittles you. Whatever the situation don't allow another person to take you over entirely.

If you are depressed refuse to allow the depression to take you over completely, or to dictate the colour and direction of your life.

At all times explore, experiment and discuss but avoid playing power and control games with others. This may occur when a woman wishes to attract male interest but is too insecure and uncertain to flirt or be direct. She may attract his attention and then look through him or confuse the situation by looking away and ignoring him.

Such games are usually infantile in origin, often linked to strong feelings of jealousy and more about power politics than making contact. They can lead to paranoid feelings of being looked at and observed by others, which is unsettling and adds to tension and a heightened imaginative state.

Keep your body language and your relationships direct and simple. Maintain contact with the more mature sides of your personality and value the unique individual you are.

THE LONELINESS OF THE LONG DISTANCE RUNNER

If you are feeling agitated and restless, unable to relax, with strong impulses to run out of the house, let your partner know and warn him or a friend what you want to do. In this way if you do need to run out, someone can accompany you for company and safety.

Try to anticipate when this is going to happen and what triggers any severe feelings of panic, anxiety and restlessness. Talk through with your partner why the feelings have erupted at this time. It may be linked to specific fear, a new situation, rivalry or jealousy, sometimes heightened sexuality.

Make your running creative, with an aim and a reason. When the feelings are less intense, relax and walk or run with your partner. Look, visit, photograph and enjoy. Avoid stimulants, such as strong coffee and tea, which will give you a 'high' at a time when you need to relax.

If you hear voices telling you what to do and where to go or feel others are directing your thoughts, try to see these as reflecting a part of you which has become displaced and lost. Make every attempt to link back to them and be prepared to spend time doing this. Bring all aspects of your thoughts and feelings to the surface as you work at the internal split.

As you walk or run, release the tensions and let go of anxiety, fears and any compulsive thoughts. Try to express yourself openly, without holding back or being judgmental and self-critical.

FOOT LOOSE

Feeling restless and irritable may be your way of expressing a frightened and damaged part of yourself. It is important to express those aspects of yourself as well as any part of you which has been denied or repressed.

Any healing attempt to release a repressed or a deprived part of you, which has been kept under strict control and felt to be unacceptable or damaging, will inevitably cause you some anxiety. Impulses to harm yourself can be an attempt to hide or block the healing process, fearing failure or rejection.

A resurgence of childhood memories can lead to depression and a sense that everything is futile and pointless. It is important to forge links with all aspects of your mind, including a more dynamic, healthy you.

Allow your feelings to emerge, including those of anxiety and fear and find words to express them. Look at your dreams for clues and share these with your partner. A major change in your life - a wedding, house-move, holiday, flight, or hospital admission to have a baby - may cause insecurity, triggering infantile feelings and fears of abandonment or breaking the umbilical tie. Leaving home even for a short period, may equate with a break from security.

Clarify what is happening and avoid blocking the expression of new and emerging aspects of yourself. These are sometimes initially expressed as anxiety and fear but also reflect positive moves towards maturity, growth and integration. Keep it simple.

'MI5'

Occasionally, the 'blues' becomes more severe and a mum experiences a state of turmoil. This may provoke quite desperate feelings: a persecuted state of mind, hearing voices, believing actions and comments are directed at her, others are scheming or plotting.

In order to reach a better understanding of those parts of your mind which are locked into a persecuted mode of thinking, look at any areas where you have a grudge, or feel preoccupied with a sense of injustice and would like to take revenge on those who have hurt or rejected you. Often this occurred in childhood and involved another member of the family, perhaps an older sister was more favoured or a brother could do no wrong.

For some the emotional fire is centred on more recent events: passed over for promotion, cheated by a colleague, redundancy, an accident which left you scarred or damaged. This inner feud, either recent or remote, usually involves enraged basic feelings, hurt pride, phantasies of revenge and sometimes plans to put these into action. Feelings of failure or inferiority may also be at the root of the persecutory feelings or a need to be looked at and the centre of attention.

Strengthen contact with the healthy aspects of your mind. Quite simple things - listening and helping others, poetry, walking in the forest or just hugging a tree, are all helpful. Maximise trust, sharing and communication and don't brood over old conflict situations.

Remain simple and focused and try to acknowledge, accept and care for all aspect of your feelings.

A LIVING NIGHTMARE

If you are frightened by some nameless threat or sense of doom, share the panic feelings with your family and friends. This will bring some reality and logic back into the situation. Often the fear is that the feelings and needs will be too strong and lead to rejection.

Make a link between the feelings and the situation which triggered the fears. If you have experienced them in the past, look back to the reasons for the first attack. Are there any links between then and the pressures and events which caused a recent problem to occur now?

Accept your feelings but don't allow them to devour your mind or to take over. At the same time avoid blocking or denying their existence. Accept the feelings but don't be manipulated and dictated by them. Talk back, argue, be even more persuasive and determined than the impulses or illogical thoughts. They can only derive their determination and force from your inner fears and drive. Treat them as guests but don't allow them to outstay their welcome or be taken in by them. Don't take them too seriously and they will eventually pack their bags and go. Avoid secrecy at all times.

Don't stay alone in a desperate situation, get help immediately. Practice relaxation at times of turmoil and find ways to loosen-up the problems.

The expression of a storm of feelings often heralds a break-through. Don't panic, stay in touch with yourself and find a simple, calmer, more mature you to reassure yourself and to stay centred. This will help you maintain a more cohesive whole.

INTERACTION SHEET 5
A REVIEW OF YOUR SYMPTOMS
date

Write down in order of importance, your main symptoms of the 'blues'. How do your present symptoms compare with those recorded on Interactive sheet 1?

In this way, you can compare your symptoms and any progress made.

1.

2.

3.

4.

Keep it accurate, simple and to the point. If necessary, discuss with your partner.

PORT IN A STORM

If you are isolated, desperate, or suicidal with no one to confide or trust in, ring the Samaritans. Talk to one of their helpers who will help to put your feelings back into perspective. Work at ways of taking positive action. Isolating yourself can be an attempt to defeat your best attempts at cure. It can also delay your ability to make changes, find solutions and resolve problems.

Make contact with a healthy part of you. Try to do ordinary things like going for a walk. Ignore the feelings for a time and find ways to limit their attempt to build up to a point where they dominate and take over. Stay relaxed, maintain your social contacts and whenever possible, make new friends. Listen to their concerns, feelings and needs and talk about your own thoughts and ideas but also talk about any odd or peculiar things which seem to be happening to you. Others may have been there too and may recognize the feelings. It is always helpful to know how others have coped and worked through similar emotions to reach a greater health and strength.

Don't expect immediate answers, the problem has probably taken months if not years to develop and will take time to resolve. Use the time to evolve and develop, making positive changes, improving the quality of your life, restoring and creating a new depth to your communications, relationships and life-style. Despite the problems keep moving ahead and find shifts and solutions to begin the process of change and renewal.

Reverse the process of isolation by taking positive action. Don't live in a submarine. Keep it simple.

MUM THERAPIST

date

The following short exercises are designed to help you think about a typical mum with the 'blues', from an outsider point of view. Imagine you are the therapist to each of the mums described and write down three key things she should think about and put into action.

A mum lives in a comfortable urban environment. She is unhappy and comes from a background where she was stifled and spoiled. She dislikes the noise and pollution of the city and longs for the country.

1.

2.

3.

Another mum, lives in an isolated rural situation. There are severe financial restrictions and she is without a car during the day, as her husband needs it to travel to work. She misses the bustle of the inner city where she spent her early childhood.

1.

2.

3.

An Asian mum lives with her in-laws. Her husband works away and she only sees him at weekends. She isn't allowed to visit her family and if she were to leave her husband it would be seen as a disgrace. Her mother-in-law bullies her and she has little personal money.

1.

2.

3.

The fourth mum is yourself. Deal with your problems from a therapist point of view. Look at the essentials and make suggestions to improve them.

1.

2.

3.

Help each mum think more creatively and laterally, taking a broader, more holistic approach to her problem solving. Help her understand that seeing difficulties through a narrow slit or from a narrow viewpoint distorts them and makes it harder for her. A simple, natural and direct approach is best.

THERAPY

If symptoms persist and you are not making the headway you had hoped for, you may benefit from a period of focused counselling or psychotherapy.

Therapy implies a working relationship with another person, usually a trained counsellor or therapist. The therapist listens and gives their uninvolved impressions of what is happening, the 'dynamics' of the problem, supporting you to make changes within your feelings and attitudes. The therapist acts as a facilitator or enabler, on your side but able to disagree and help you see things from a new, less self-destructive viewpoint.

Shifts and changes of attitude ought to make you feel stronger and better. But if you still feel there is an underlying problem in your job or relationship, you may need to make changes there too.

Where there have been problems in the past, therapy allows you to open up these areas with more openness and dialogue, freeing more relaxed attitudes.

The relationship and trust you are able to develop with your therapist is key to the success of the whole thing. If it doesn't seem to be working or moving, consider a change of therapist or an entirely different approach. Avoid continuing for long periods with a therapy which is going nowhere.

Be simple, frank and open with your therapist. If it is not working then change it. Only work with a person you find sympathetic, can relate to and communicate with.

PARTNERS

This section is written for men who find it difficult to know how to respond and what to do when their partner is low and 'fed up'.

The usual problem is a failure to listen and allow sufficient time for feelings to emerge or a tendency to take a rigid and narrow point of view. The partner may feel he cannot cope with tears or gets irritable, panics and takes flight. This is a lost opportunity to make changes or stop things getting worse.

What is needed is not usually complicated or particularly difficult. It is always essential: to give support and not to pass judgement, to plan for regular breaks, to help more with the children and when there is a new baby, to be less hard on the step-kids or a child who is 'difficult', challenging and provocative.

Once the partner understands what is required and it is within his capabilities, he can slow down and develop more confidence. He is then able to be more relaxed and open, communicating this to the mum and other members of the family.

When the partner is less irritable, happier and more at peace with himself, the mum can also improve because a blockage has been released. Each of you might want to consider asking :-
What have I discussed with my partner?
Have I been direct and honest?
What more can I do to help her with ?
What more can I do to help him with?
Keep your approach direct and simple.

I GOT - DELAYED

If your partner is upset and cries don't hide away or storm out. Try to understand her needs. Avoid seeing tears as a threat and another attempt to manipulate you. Don't condemn her for the expression of her genuine needs for time and attention. These are bound to be much more intensive at times of exhaustion and despair.

Unless they are a macho display or linked to male virility, men are not usually good at showing feelings and tend to hide or deny them. There is a tendency to stifle and deny all other feelings including sadness and need. Many men cannot cope or feel threatened by such feelings. Women are much more confident at showing feelings and over the years have shared tears and feeling with their family and female friends and been able to express emotions and feelings at period times.

Your relationship will benefit if both partners allow their emotions to be shown and shared. At times of disappointment and loss avoid denial of your own feelings of sadness and despair.

Show and share your emotions and become more open with them. You will also gain in confidence and develop a better understanding of the feelings and needs of your partner.

Listen more and talk less but listen actively and in an involved way. Taking flight from feelings will isolate and weaken you in the long run. Keep it simple throughout.

NOT SO GLORIOUS BEER

She probably requires more than a can of beer and another night of sport on the box to cheer her up. Learn about the real needs and feelings of your partner and how these link up with the past, her experiences as a child and adolescent, the joys and fears these engendered.

Broaden and share your activities and interests and talk more about them. If you enjoy a drink at the local and a game of soccer that's fine but also take on new and joint projects which include her and the children, sometimes just the two of you.

If she enjoys your sport and wants to come along, support and participate, she may also need to spend some time alone with you, to talk, share and just to cuddle up. Make sure that you are being open with her and not avoiding her needs for support, commitment, closeness and sharing.

Find out what her interests are and be there with her some of the time. Soften and expand any narrow or rigid attitudes. Make changes and enjoy new things. Try a different sport or restaurant you both enjoy. You can still support your local club and have a drink as well but keep your intake sensible and moderate.

Make sure she knows that you love her and still care. Be prepared to talk about and share your own childhood experiences and how this has affected you. Listen and share her feelings, present needs and past experiences.

PUNCH AND JUDY

If your partner is depressed give her more time and not less. Listen to what is upsetting her. She may find it difficult or takes time to express herself in depth, frightened of your reactions, becoming defensive, snappy, or 'up tight' because this was her experience in the past when she felt vulnerable and terrified.

Withdrawal and getting depressed may have been her way of coping in the past and it takes confidence to evolve a new way for dealing with fear, panic and uncertainty.

Stay cool at all times and keep your alcohol low to nil, especially if you have a tendency to become violent. Make contact with a quiet and calm, reasonable side of you which is prepared to listen, make changes and to compromise. Find new ways to show your caring and interest. Develop new interests and new friends and encourage her to do likewise. Be as open as possible and involve her in what you are doing and your main goals and projects. Talk and share with her and learn from each other. Her suggestions and ideas, as well as your own, may be very helpful and valuable.

If you do lose your cool apologise as soon as possible and explain how and why it happened. Keep working on expressing your feelings without losing control or allowing them to erupt.

At all times avoid getting irritable, threatening or violent as this will only confirm her worst fears. Don't be afraid to keep your ideas and comments simple and to the point.

GONE TO MOTHER

If there is a separation and she goes back to the family or a friend, go along, see her, listen and talk. Don't just sit passively and make promises to make amends, use the opportunity to make a clear statement of your feelings at the time of the break up, what led up to it and why it erupted. Let her know clearly how you have been feeling and how much you miss and need her.

In order to give yourself more understanding, as well as your partner, use the separation to make contact with your feelings and to bring them more into the open. Making a change in the way you express your emotions will also improve the quality of your communications.

Make a time to see her again. Take her out, talk and explain that she can come back when and if she feels happy to do so. Clarify together what are her problems and needs and how you can give the extra backing and support she needs to feel secure and happy.

Make certain she feels valued, wanted and cared for. Discuss calmly why she has felt the need to distance herself and plan together the changes needed to improve matters in the future.

Pressurising her or imposing a time-table for her to return is not helpful. She must feel ready and confident to do so. This will take time, according to the depth of the recent problem, what has occurred in the past and the trust as well as hurts and splits which exist between you.

Stay straightforward and simple.

Take the children out and give her a break. This will help both of you and the kids will enjoy the time spent with you and the contact. Make sure you listen to their needs, relating to them at their level and giving them the time and space they need to explore, discuss and share.

Avoid becoming irritable when they inevitably become noisy, undisciplined, excited, boisterous and hungry. If they don't tend to misbehave you may be over-strict with them, or they are fearful and in awe of you. This would indicate the need to give them more time and to rebuild their confidence as well as that of your partner.

Make arrangements for a day or a weekend away. It need not be expensive. The simple things in life: a day exploring on the cliffs, a picnic at the seaside, a ramble in the woods are not expensive. If you are not taking the children - help sort out who will baby-sit them when you are away.

Be more supportive and ask her how you can routinely help with the day-to-day chores. Share the routines and show her that you enjoy being with her and want to help and support her. She may also want to share some of your chores and interests and to lend a hand. Make sure she feels welcome and wanted and be prepared for a few surprises and to learn some new ideas, suggestions and shortcuts from her feminine intuitive skills.

When she shows ability and skills in your area, as well as her own, don't reject her or immediately become irritable.

VACATION

Have a family holiday each year and plan it with her and the children. Let them also be actively involved and help with the planning. Vary the resort and also the type of holiday.

Alcohol on vacation or during the flights is a common cause of family problems. It sets a bad example to the children and it is far healthier to drink water or juices in flight to combat dehydration rather than alcohol.

Make the holiday interesting and relaxing for her. Don't always go to the same beach or centre you personally choose, make it a shared initiative. If the children want to stay in the pool for the whole day and don't want to visit, negotiate with them, planning in advance the time away and when you will get back.

If you have young children ensure trips to historical sites, museums or galleries are kept short but do some background research and share this with them. Your involvement and enthusiasm will make it more interesting for them but make sure they also know at what time they will be back at the pool or beach to meet their friends. They will also be happier if they know a snack or meal treat is included in any outing.

If you want to sun and sleep, read by the pool, with long lazy days and no cultural pursuits, ensure this also suits your partner. Make some time for walking, cycling and the occasional informative trip.

Not just on holiday but throughout the year, keep your alcohol intake down to reasonable levels.

STROLLING

Go for regular walks or bike rides together. Talk but also create a space to be quiet and still in. At times leave the kids at home, relax and just enjoy each other's company.

Walk at a pace you can both comfortably sustain and enjoy. You are not running a race or training for the Olympics. Exercise is good for you but don't make it damaging, excessive, prolonged or punishing.

Vary your walking, exploring new areas and pathways. Slowly build up your stamina, increasing the distance you walk and provided you both enjoy it, plan a walking, camping or trekking holiday. Stretching and warm ups are essential before any form of exercise, especially long uphill climbs or walks on uneven terrain. Make sure it is not too hard for young children if they are coming along.

Try walking in a group and if you enjoy a more organised experience, join them regularly and make new friends with other hikers.

Plan your walks for looking at nature and enjoying the countryside as well as fitness and health. Ensure you have the best supportive footwear and are also using the latest technology clothing. In this way you will stay comfortable and minimise any damage to your joints. Always walk in areas where security is not an issue and if necessary get professional advice.

Avoid getting into arguments, blaming her, excusing yourself, or point-scoring.

CHEZ MAXIM'S

Take her out and give her a break from preparing meals and washing-up. Make it a surprise but ensure she has enough time to organise her hair and make-up.

You may both need to change your routines and to lighten your mood after a demanding, tiring day. If you eat out regularly make sure you vary it. Avoid watching television when you eat and use the meal time to eat slowly, relax, talk and share. Keep the ideas flowing. Try to participate in your partner's workload. If you feel jaded and exhausted she may have had an even more tiring day. Don't just sit there sullen, sulking and withdrawn.

Find different things to do and vary the places you visit and both enjoy. Be prepared to compromise and to travel but don't make every trip a burden because of the stress vibes you bring to it. Combine a meal out with the theatre, show, or club. Make sure it is not only your choice and she also wants to be there.

Energise and invigorate your relationship and give it more hope and momentum. Too often the relationship has lost its direction. Make it a priority but make sure you are giving it enough time and space. Don't expect changes to occur overnight. You are looking for a fundamental change in your relationship where you can think laterally, creatively and above all, jointly and together.

Don't get irritable if she takes longer than you to get ready. Stay cool and let her do things in her time. If you arrive a little late, so what.

SATURDAY NIGHT

Tell her you care and hold her. According to both your tastes take her to a club or dance, or somewhere quiet that you would both find relaxing and enjoyable.

Keep your sexuality flexible by varying your approach, talking, looking, stroking and not rushing. It may not be necessary to have sex all night, she may prefer less frequently rather than more. Anticipate that her female cycle and hormone levels will have some input into her libidinal appetite and it will differ from your own masculine arousal patterns.

Your partner may not be able to achieve a full orgasm after the birth because of pain and fear, or because she is too tired. Don't insist on intercourse if she is not in the mood. Avoid having prolonged sex after a new baby or anything which causes discomfort or pain.

Saturday night should not be an all or nothing thing, the only night when you go out or have sex. Vary the times when you are intimate, the things you do and how you do them.

Find a new, easy, relaxed and enjoyable approach to sex, closeness, intimacy, sharing and life.

Avoid making sex the be all and end all of life. Don't just have sex, turn over and sleep or snore. Talk to her and share more of yourself. Make plans together for your joint future and include her in each planning stage.

SUPPORT

Give her backing and support at all levels, especially when there is a new baby or very young children. A partner may opt out of closeness because he feels threatened, fearing a demand for immediate solutions to problems which he knows have worried the mum for months and have not been fully talked through.

Lack of communication and a failure to share are the prime culprits for an impasse within the couple. If her energy levels are low or depleted, rather than complaining or making demands the partner needs to be there with her, to share and give a hand.

Just taking an interest and listening are often most important. The fact that you have made the time to be involved means she feels more valued. You don't have to be there all the time but it does help if you both share any grinding chores in the evening and at weekends. If she is tired and you are dithering she will probably snap and be sharp. You may take on the role of the hurt innocent victim, rather than seeing how you provoked her in the first place. This may end in tears and another row.

Aim for spontaneity and simplicity and avoid rigid patterns of behaviour, the predictable and the expected. Be prepared to experiment and improvise. Ask your partner to help you recognize your patterns of sameness and try to vary them.

Remember, the basic psychological human needs are for quite simple things: support, listening, sharing, to be valued and a cuddle.

STEP KIDS

If you have been married before and brought the kids with you there are bound to be divisions, tensions and tears, as everyone fights to be 'top dog'. There will also be disciplinary problems to agree on and rules will have to be established. The kids will test you both to the limit and at times blame your partner for being unreasonable, punitive and insensitive.

Children will always exploit any areas of inconsistency or weakness and it is essential to agree an overall style and approach to parenting, discipline and the management of emotional problems which are bound to surface at sometime. Every day give some individual time to each child, so that he or she feels they are getting that little bit extra and knows they are loved, special and valued.

At some point they will try to create a split, in order to get you back in their camp and under their control. You will need all your communicative and diplomatic skills, sense of humour and capacity to work together as a couple to keep the ship afloat. If mum has time to be depressed in this situation she will be stretched, as the pressures call for even greater team work.

The 'difficult' child is usually asking for love and attention in the only way he knows but everyone else in the family is also fighting for a piece of the 'loved and valued' cake, each in his or her individual way.

It is hard work, beset with demands and problems but very rewarding and well worth the effort. Play it cool and keep it simple.

INTERACTIVE SHEET FOR PARTNERS 1.
date
What more can I do to help her with:-

Keep it simple and ensure you have been open and honest.

INTERACTIVE SHEET FOR PARTNERS 2.
date
What more can I do to help him with:-.

**Keep it simple and ensure you have been open and
honest.**

MATURE MUMS

It is not only young mums with babies and small children who become depressed. Mature mums also have babies and can get even more tired and run down than young ones.

Mums also feel that with aging life becomes more difficult and complicated. It is easy to lose confidence and if she has problems with her partner she may increasingly depend on a good relationship with her children and grandchildren. All may go smoothly and well, as long as there are no major changes or problems but if a breakdown of her marriage occurs, or she loses her husband from an accident or illness, it can be devastating.

If she is not able to make adjustments and changes this may lead to tension and the 'blues'. A mature mum may not always find it easy to make the changes which are necessary to rebuild confidence. She may need to heal a breakdown in her own marriage, or divorce and start a new relationship. It takes time and energy to build and project a confident and attractive image. If she is planning to marry again and have another family she may feel under pressure by time and the number of fertile eggs left before the menopause.

Make the effort, give yourself the time and the opportunity for change to occur. Don't exhaust yourself under a mountain of unnecessary chores or endless worrying about something that has not happened.

DIVORCE

If the children divorce and the mum has become fond of her ex-son or daughter-in-law, or there are grandchildren, this can be an especially painful time.

She may be concerned about hurts to both parties, how much the children are suffering or feel both acted unreasonably and that divorce is no answer to their problems.

A wife may blame her mother-in-law for all the problems of the marriage and feel she interfered and took sides or was an undermining influence.

Resentful feelings may be very strong if she feels her mother-in-law is trying to influence her husband, weakening her position and authority or threatening to tie the son to her apron-strings and keep him a child.

Find a different way to think about your life and your problems. Look at the alternatives and the changes you are able to make rather than those you cannot. Expand and develop them.

If problems occur, build bridges and maintain contacts and communication. Be prepared to listen, swallow your pride and admit you have made mistakes.

PAST REGRETS

If the mature mum has divorced she may regret the break-up of her marriage, missing the company even if caring was minimal towards the end. If she is on her own this may intensify loneliness and despair. Even if the children are attentive she can still feel they are no substitute for a husband or mature male companion.

If there have been several previous marriages and divorces she may still feel attached to a previous husband, think about him and miss him. A problem may also occur if the marriage seemed happy, with no obvious problems or rows and there was no clear explanation as to why the relationship ended.

A static, closed state of mind linked to an unhappy past will cause depression. Allow yourself to live and grow in the present, widening your interests and learn to value yourself more. Becoming more involved with new interests, new contacts and new friends will help you. Use the past as a springboard into the present and the future, rather than a barrier to change and renewal.

Try to make a break with the past and move on to new friendships and interests in the present. Don't hang on to the past because of insecurity or the past is familiar and known. You will gain and grow far more by moving on to different areas and making new friends and contacts in the present. Pain, disappointment and hurt do not necessarily lead to suffering and resentment, they can also be a blessing and lead to a deeper appreciation and understanding, a deeper love and capacity to bond.

MY DARLING DAUGHTER

As a mum gets older she may feel more vulnerable, unsure of herself and increasingly dependent. This dependent relationship is made more intense if the mum is depressed and on her own.

See your daughter and any grandchildren regularly but don't impose your ideals and values on them. Make sure you are not dominated by a morbid side of yourself which has never been fully resolved and may often date from childhood.

Problems in infancy can often affect the whole of your life and an experience of loss or rejection at that time is a common cause of depression in later years. If this does apply to you, ask yourself if you have truly moved on since that time and if there is any reason e.g. a sick and elderly dependent relative, which prevents you from healing and freeing yourself from the past and moving on into a new and healthier you.

If there is a recurrent emotional problem, for instance ambivalent feelings or outbursts of anger, ensure that you are not avoiding problems in the present by blaming or gnawing away at yourself. Find ways to confront and resolve what has happened and release any feelings associated with that time. Make it a priority to find ways to liberate yourself and to renew yourself.

Build confidence by going out more, making new friends, joining a group and planning holidays with friends. Try to expand your areas of interest and enjoyment. At all times keep moving forward and maintain physical fitness by regular exercise.

DAUGHTER-IN-LAW

Problems often occur when the mature mum does not approve of the partner her child chooses. She may feel he or she is unsuitable, doesn't have money, savings, position or security, has been divorced, doesn't share the same faith, comes from a different social and educational background, is too old or young, lacks robust health or shares different aims and values from herself.

In some areas the mum may have remained a child and not been able to separate herself from the ideals and values of her own parents which were imposed on her. For this reason she finds it difficult to relinquish controls and finds reassurance by imposing narrow value judgments on herself and her family. Sameness is what matters and reassures her, rather than the unknown and the unpredictable which she finds frightening rather than challenging. This kind of controlling behaviour does not however reassure the young mum and is quickly seen through and tends to make her withdraw.

Stop pre-judging others, trying to live their lives for them. Cut the umbilical cord. Accept that this may not be your ideal choice of partner but you will benefit by being fair, open-minded and not pressurising her or being so judgmental. Give more time to getting to know your daughter-in-law and to exchange feelings and ideas. She will inevitably have a totally different approach from your more traditional one, but with time and patience you may end up liking each other.

WIDOW SPIDER

If the mature mum, loses her husband, she may feel quite at sea, finding it difficult to cope with the loss and the mourning and unsure of herself afterwards. This may increase dependency feelings and infantile attitudes of fear and panic. For others it is the reverse and after the period of mourning is briefly over, the mum positively blossoms and goes from strength to strength.

Much depends on the mum's intrinsic strength, her previous early experiences and her ability to re-new and adapt to changing circumstances.

Stop attacking and devaluing yourself or taking flight from renewal and making a commitment to the present. Try to perceive why you are depressed and the main areas where you have lost confidence. Discuss the problem with your friends and family and try to understand how they see it and if they can come up with any suggestions or solutions. Don't immediately write these off as non-starters but try them and think them through.

Avoid locking yourself into a mood of blank despair. If you are feeling angry and disappointed about life let the feelings come to the surface and have life. Use the energy of these feelings positively and stay with them. Let the feelings fire you but not to take you over in an obsessional or compulsive way. Keep an open, flexible mind at all times, prepared to experiment, explore and to be more daring.

Avoid isolating yourself and withdrawing. Don't let pride or fear keep you lonely and in isolation.

LONELY MUM

After a period of acute mourning is over, if her needs are not met, the mature mum may feel neglected or redundant. If feelings of depression increase she may feel her children show no real care or interest because she is old, or no longer has a role of any importance.

If there is insufficient regular contact for her needs and to reassure her, she can feel her daughter-in-law is critical and hostile, makes no real attempt to understand her or become a friend. If resentful feelings intensify she may suspect her daughter-in-law is against her, deliberately alienating her son and grandchildren from her or even plotting against her.

Stop feeling sorry for yourself, using your age or state of health as a defence against change. Renew your attitudes and outlook on life. Getting fit physically and emotionally will re-energise you and improve your outlook. It is never too late to take up a new interest and meet a new group of friends. Don't bury your head in the sand or in your hands. Make sure that you are not critical or hostile towards change rather than welcoming it as healthy and inevitable.

Improve your sense of self-esteem and self-value by doing something you have wanted to do but always put off. It can be anything but make sure it is something you are going to enjoy and will give you satisfaction.

Try to express any feelings of resentment and hostility which you have and talk them through with your friends and also the family. Don't hold grudges or keep them secret.

MARRIAGE WITHOUT ISSUE

The mature mum may become depressed because she feels the young couple put security and finance before having a family. She may fear she will die before they have children and will never see her grandchildren. If she puts pressure on the couple they can resent this or feel emotionally blackmailed and withdraw themselves from her. All of this increases her sense of isolation, failure and frustration.

Whatever your age avoid only seeing life in terms of your own personal stereotypes, standards and ideals. This implies a rigid position which is not in your best interests or those of the couple.

A mature mum may feel depressed or threatened because she perceives an absence of children and of direct lineage as a failure to create a process which carries her name and her genes. The absence of a family comes to symbolise an ending and is more about her fear of dying and the aging process than about life and creating.

Avoid imposing values and count your blessings. Enjoy what you have rather than what you don't and try not to only think negatively, find fault or to be dissatisfied. Think on a larger and different scale and clarify how one idea relates to another and leads to change.

Avoid seeing the life-style and ambitions of your children through your eyes and needs. They also have their own agenda. You may not always agree but try to understand it and learn to identify with their hopes and joys.

MUM ON HER OWN

Problems sometimes occur because the mature mum needs some extra support but does not like to admit she feels lonely and frightened. She may have few friends and becomes too dependent on family visits. This can cause a pressure situation to develop and a tendency for the children to distance themselves, aggravating her depression. In part this may be because they are unsure how best to help her.

Try not to be so dependent on the children and grandchildren or the family. Make new friends as well as retaining links with old ones. Maintain the contact by telephone, e-mail, writing, visits and holidays. Go out each day. Do something. See someone. Talk to and show an interest in another person and keep your body and mind alive, active and expanding.

Aim for a deeper meaning to your relationships. Never be frightened to ask questions, however simple or to search for new insights, meanings and understanding with your partner. Ask, think, seek and expand.

Don't use age as a defence against change, renewal and modernisation of your ideas and understanding.

Let yourself flow and be at peace with yourself as you do so.

Be prepared to express your feelings and needs. Don't hide them away or put on a facade if you are feeling 'down'. Make sure the family knows when you are depressed and always confide in a friend.

MY SON, MY SON

If in the early years the mum divorced, or was rigid and over-strict with the children, in later years they may resent this and punish her by withholding care, affection and interest.

This creates a difficult relationship for the mum which she may not easily understand and finds hard to accept. The son or daughter-in-law may blame the mum for failings in their own relationship, looking for a scapegoat to take responsibility for the lack of a more caring, imaginative approach to marriage.

Accept that being rejected or ignored at times is part of life. Don't complain or indulge in self pity. It is healthier to accept that at times you are capable of being vicious in your thinking rather than trying to suppress it. This may make you feel better and the mischievous thoughts will get you out of the role of always being wronged and the victim who is rejected. In your inner mind feel free to do some of the rejecting and blaming too and don't feel guilty about it. You are allowed to have ambivalent feelings about your family however much you love them. It is inevitable that you will apportion feelings in segments and at times someone will be seen as generous and kind, someone else as lazy, selfish and a bitch. Get the feelings out, the good and the bad, then forget them and get on with living.

Remain calm and on an even keel. Be prepared to talk things through from the past when they come up in conversation. Don't be surprised or wrong-footed by powerful emotions which emerge on all sides, including those from yourself.

INTERACTIVE SHEET 6.   THE OUTCOME
date
**Write down any new ideas and feelings which have
been stimulated by reading the book. Keep your
comments as original and personal to you as
possible.**

1.

2.

3.

4.

Always keep your thoughts and comments simple and succinct.

MUM AND HER MUM

To a large extent, all mums are dependent on their own mum for their identity and a role model. A mum plays a key part in the attitudes a daughter adapts towards her sexuality and femininity. The way her first period is dealt with, first steps towards clothes, make-up, hair style, boy friends and sex are all key issues for the teenager and the degree of confidence she develops in later year as a mum herself.

If from the start mum keeps the shutters down, is disapproving or doesn't talk about such things with her daughter, including her own problems and experiences, this creates a burden for the young budding woman, cramping her freedom of expression and style.

Make sure you are open and honest. Deal with any question about the female body, its cycle and functioning, love and sex in a very direct way. Be prepared to deal with any questions which your daughter, grandchild or your own mum throws at you, answering at a level they can understand and relate to. Often the most important thing is not what is actually asked or your reply but the way you say it and how frank, easy and unfazed you are but treat all aspects of life in the same way, including any provocative questions from your sons or partner.

If the mature mum is supportive and understanding this reinforces her daughter's femininity and builds confidence. This helps the future mum to be more relaxed with her sexuality throughout life and she will also approach motherhood in a more easy, happy way.

ALTERNATIVE THERAPY

SUSTAINING HOMOEOPATHY

If you are pregnant or there is a possibility that you might be or if you are nursing a young baby, it is of the utmost importance to be extremely cautious about what supplements, over-the-counter drugs, prescribed medicines or herbal remedies you put into your system at this time. During the early developmental stages the young foetus is extremely vulnerable. Make sure you are well-informed about the possible risks of atomizers, perfume sprays and sun screens. You may also want to minimize the use of any synthetic additives and the same applies when you are breast-feeding. In a word, keep it simple and natural.

I recommend homoeopathy as one of the safest and best forms of alternative or complementary medicine for mums. It is widely used and without risk if you are pregnant or breast-feeding. It is also perfectly safe to use for babies and young children and over many years it has been shown to work well and effectively.

KALI PHOS. 6c (Potassium phosphate)
One of the best remedies for states of fatigue, exhaustion and anxiety.
AC. PHOS. 6c (Phosphoric acid)
Another excellent remedy, especially for states of complete exhaustion and burn-out.
NUX MOSCHATA 6c (Nutmeg)
Useful where drowsiness is associated with fatigue and a dry throat. The patient tends to feel chilly and bloated with indigestion problems.

THINK HOMOEOPATHY

If prepared correctly, by a process of serial dilution and succussion (vigorous shaking to dynamise the remedy), the homoeopathic remedies or potencies contain the vital energy of the original substance and no detectable amounts of the original herb or mineral material. For this reason they can be taken without risk.

CHINA 6c (Peruvian bark or Cinchona officinalis)

A useful remedy for persistent states of fatigue and where the vital reserves of the mum have been depleted.

There is a flat, drowsy state of mind, usually due to lack of rest and the mum having been continuously on the go for a period of weeks or months. She feels at the end of her tether and is still tired after a sleep or rest period. The mum feels as if she needs to sleep for a month. Digestive discomfort is common and all her complaints are very variable but quickly worse for any effort because she has no reserves and is overtired.

See yourself on a journey of change, learning and experience. Ask yourself: Why did I say it in that way? Why was I so sharp? Why was I swamped by those emotions? Why did I react in such a hard, rejecting way? What made me talk to him like that? Be honest with yourself.

A depressed state of mind will weaken and exhaust you. At all times, try to retain contact with a healthy positive side of you which will help uplift you. Be emphatic and don't let negative feelings totally take over.

GENTLE HOMOEOPATHY

If you are frequently tearful, with changes in emotion and mood, consider trying homoeopathy as a viable alternative approach. At the same time, try to learn more about the method and why it is so effective.

PULSATILLA 6c (Wind flower)

This deep acting remedy is indicated for the mum who feels tired, anxious and tearful. Changeable in mood, she is anxious and fearful, at other times irritable, shy or lacking in confidence. Typically the mum prefers being in the fresh air and cool conditions, the windows open and feels better in the springtime and for being outdoors but she usually avoids the sun and prefers to sit in areas of dappled shade. She languishes in close stuffy, airless situations. Thirst is usually absent and nasal or sinus problems are common. Fatty foods are not well tolerated and indigestion is a common problem.

Allow for variations within your feelings and also your partner. Don't expect to be constant and on an even keel all of the time. There are bound to be variations in your mood, feelings and behaviour.

Step outside your problems and look at them from a different perspective. Once you develop a new point of view there is a new understanding, you have made a shift and a significant change has occurred.

Pack up your troubles for the day and leave your worries behind you. Assert a new more positive you. Build strength and confidence but also allow concern for others to emerge.

SOOTHING HOMOEOPATHY

A mum can ache at the end of the day and feel bruised or shattered psychologically. She is often overtired, her sleep is disturbed and there is just too much to do.

ARNICA 6c (Fall Kraut)

This is a marvellous homoeopathic plant remedy which acts on the mind and the body for bruised weariness. It is excellent both before and after the delivery and can safely be used for an aching sense of fatigue. The mum is often tense, her skin hypersensitive and this makes the bed feel hard or uncomfortable.

Arnica is a remedy for apprehension, being accident prone and lacking drive and energy reserves. It is indicated when the mum feels apprehensive or vulnerable and is anxious to avoid close contacts and lacks confidence. She is usually both tired and apathetic and has never fully recovered from the birth or sometimes an acute shock, disappointment or trauma.

Brain-storm any area where you feel blocked. Let the ideas and feelings just flow out of you. Look at the reasonable, attainable ideas but also look at the unattainable ones. Work out ways to make the latter become a reachable option. Challenge your imagination. Stretch yourself psychologically. Find ways to make the unachievable an achievable reality.

Consider homoeopathy as a primary (first-line) treatment for the family, rather than a secondary back-up approach only used after conventional drugs have failed.

DEEP ACTING HOMOEOPATHY

Problems of jealousy, resentment and anger are not uncommon for a mum who is depressed and they may cause severe anxiety and guilt feelings.

LACHESIS 6c (Bushmaster snake venom)

This important remedy is of especial value for hormonal disturbances and when there is a very disturbed state of mind. The mum is restless, self-conscious and often lacks confidence and energy. She has a tendency to be over-talkative, prone to feeling jealous and angry, disliking tight fitting clothing of any description.

She tends to feel exhausted and is typically worse if she wakes up during the night or in the morning after sleep. Left-sided discomfort is a feature, either in the throat or in one limb. A blotchy face, purple skin marks or bruises and discolourations are a feature, linked to a tendency to bleed easily.

In order to reach a more balanced position ask yourself: What am I doing with my life and what sort of person have I become? What sort of person can I be? What are my directions, priorities and goals?

If you don't understand your doctor tell him so.
If you don't understand your partner tell him now.

Avoid any therapy or medication which acts to control or suppress you. These are rarely in your interest. However disturbed your feelings and behaviour it is always preferable for these to be expressed, rather than stifled or suppressed.

IF ONLY

If your problem is one of acute grief, the sudden, traumatic loss of a loved one, you may feel responsible or blame yourself with devastating feelings of loss, anguish and despair. It may seem impossible to find a way out of the depressive mood which traps you into a perpetual low state without comfort or hope.

IGNATIA 6c (Saint Ignatia Bean)

This is an excellent and well proven remedy for a severe reaction to grief, disappointment, rejection, hurt or setback. The mum feels unable to accept what has happened or to work through the grief and return to a normal life. A wide variety of mood states may occur associated with rage, resentment, disbelief, confusion and despair.

Ignatia is indicated after an acute shock or loss with feelings of anguish, weeping and sighing, alternating with moods of rage and irritability. It is difficult to come to terms with the loss or disappointment and the mum may become withdrawn into herself, reluctant to talk. Often she is unable to sleep and wanders about the house at night, going into the room of a loved one or sitting around and waiting for him or her to return.

Accept the pain and the loss however difficult and for their sake be strong. Allow yourself a life and a future and let them live again through you. In this way they can identify with you, rather than you identifying with them (often because of guilt) as an inert and dead object or thing.

TRUST HOMOEOPATHY

Homoeopathy matches the symptom profile (the complaints and symptoms) of the whole person to the toxic symptoms of the remedy, if it were taken in its raw and undiluted form. It is then given to the patient as a potency or remedy which has been prepared by a process of serial dilution. Vigorously shaking the remedy at each stage of the dilution enhances its therapeutic action.

SEPIA 6c.(Ink of cuttle fish)

This is a deep acting remedy for severe states of fatigue. Exhaustion, nausea, irritability drag down the mum with crippling aches and pains in her back and pelvic areas. She may be indifferent to the baby and her partner and many of her deepest emotions are blocked. The mum may feel unable to cry but senses she would feel better if she could shed tears. Where the problems are severe the mum may be in a tense and disturbed emotional state, with self-destructive thoughts or impulses to harm the baby. Because of a sluggish pelvic circulation she usually feels better for any form of rapid movement, such as a brisk walk or dancing but may have to be almost dragged there before she admits there has been an improvement.

Avoid taking yourself to the limit. Learn to stop and relax before you become exhausted or over-tired. In this way you will adapt a more caring attitude to yourself which is sustaining and it will help you avoid 'burn-out' or depletion of those very important energy reserves.

SHORT FUSE

It is not uncommon for mums who are depressed to develop other more physical symptoms and indigestion and constipation are both common problems which add to a personality which is already stretched to the limit and ready to snap at the least provocation.

NUX VOMICA 6c (Poison Nut)

Many mums with the 'blues' feel cut off and exhausted. If she feels she is only just coping and not really making progress this only adds to her problems and she can panic or feel quite desperate. Irritable because she is so tired, she is ready to snap at any one who comes near her and makes a demand. She must have space around her and cannot tolerate time wasters or being hemmed in by 'stupid' questions, even sympathetic ones, which take up time and energy. At the same time she knows she is 'in a state' and too quick to anger, usually to her partner and often the children, feeling guilty about it but she is unable to control her tongue and lashes out at the least pressure or demand. She cannot tolerate foolish mistakes and is just as hard on herself if she makes an error. This is a useful remedy for tension and stress often associated with indigestion - nausea, wind, heartburn, stomach pains after eating. Constipation is another problem which adds to her discomfort.

It is always better to express any feelings of anger and irritability, rather than attempting to bottle them up but try to discuss any problem areas in a quiet, calm way and to have a dialogue about any specific problem area. If you do lose your cool you can apologise later.

BREAKING INTO PIECES

Occasionally a mum becomes much more disturbed and severely ill, unable to cope with the demands and the intensity of her feelings. An exhausting, restless state of mind may develop with impulses to destroy or damage, feeling energised and excitable, unable to sleep or rest.

HYOSCYAMUS NIGER 6c (Henbane)

This is an important plant remedy which acts directly on the brain and is indicated for very disturbed, confused, suspicious states of mind. A delusional attitude of mind may develop, sometimes with hallucination, fearing that others seek to harm her or are plotting against her. She may have impulses to destroy or damage. The mum is restless but despite being exhausted is unable to sleep. Her skin feels sensitive and she dislikes being covered, pulling the sheets off. Because of fear and a high level of muscular tension, her body makes jerky movements. She tends to dislike and is suspicious of water or the sound of running liquids.

You are as you think and perceive. Aim for a different approach and angle to your problems and the way you think about them.

It is essential to have professional help, medication and support for this kind of problem. Always consult your health visitor or doctor at an early stage, rather than delaying. Avoid isolating yourself or allowing a psychotic process (where there is a break from reality) from taking over your thoughts and mind.

Dear Reader,

I hope you have found some aspects of this little book interesting and to have some relevance to your personal problems. Not everything I have written will be applicable but some sections should strike a chord. Concentrate on these and try to expand them and make them more personal and meaningful. Only you can give them a more poignant reality.

Each section of the book is short but there is no reason why you should not enlarge it so that a section is a better 'fit' for your own personal reality. Reading alone is not a cure and if you want to make progress and changes you will need to put into operation some of the suggestions made. Resolution and cure of a problem are often directly related to your ability to make changes and at the same time to think and perceive differently, to get out of your particular 'shell' or 'rut'.

The book aims to give you a basic menu of areas to work at but it is up to you to make the choices and to build on them. You should be able to find at least two or three areas where you can make a start.

Don't just put the book down now or think about it. Keep it by you. It will only work if you use it as a working tool. Start to do something today. Begin somewhere and make it fun and enjoyable. Always remember you are unique and worth it.

Enjoy the changes and the freedom they bring.

Dr Trevor Smith.

USEFUL NATIONAL ADDRESSES TO CONTACT

The Samaritans
Helpline: 0845 7909090
A listening service to provide help in an emergency.

Meet-A-Mum Association
14, Illis Road, Croydon, CRO 2XX
Helpline: 020 8656 7318

MIND
Granta House,
15-19, Broadway, Stratford, London E15 4BQ

Association For Post Natal Depression
25, Jordan Place, Fulham, London SW6 IBE
Helpline: 020 7386 0868

The Homoeopathic Trust,
15, Clerkenwell Close, London ECIR OAA
020 7566 7800
If you don't feel confident enough to self-prescribe,
The Homoeopathic Trust will send you a list of medical
doctors in the UK who have specialised in homoeopathic
medicine.

Ainsworths Homoeopathic Pharmacy
36, New Cavendish Street, London WIM 7LH
020 7935 5330
Will supply remedies and has a mail order service.

Nelsons Homoeopathic Pharmacy
73, Duke Street, London WIM 6BY
020 7495 2404
Will supply remedies and has a mail order service.

OTHER INSIGHT PUBLICATIONS

Emotional Health (0946670 09 9)
Personal Growth & Creativity (0946670 08 0)
The Side-Effects Book (0946670 14 5)
Understanding Homoeopathy (0946670 00 5)
Talking About Homoeopathy (0946670 10 2)
Homoeopathy for Pregnancy & Nursing Mothers (0946670 17 X)
Homoeopathy for Babies & Children (0946670 15 3)
Homoeopathy for Everyday Stress Problems (0946670 19 6)
Homoeopathy for Teenagers (0946670 16 1)
Homoeopathy for Psychological Illness (0946670 20 X)
An Encyclopedia of Homoeopathy (0946670 21 8)
Guys with the Blues (0946670 22 6)
Disturbed States of Mind (0946670 21 8)